PASSING

One Woman's Pilgrimage Through Alzheimer's To Heaven

By Tana Osborn

First paperback edition November 2020
Updraft Publishing

ISBN: 978-0-9914726-6-6 (paperback)
ISBN-13: 978-0-9914726-7-3 (ebook)

www.tanaosborn.com/book-release-updates

Dedication

*This book is dedicated to all those
who have had to work through
the many heart-breaking emotions
of losing a loved one to Alzheimer's.*

Introduction

Dealing with the death of a loved one has got to be one of the hardest things we face on our current earth, but yet it is a real part of all our lives. Working as a nurse for over three decades, including hospice and as a paramedic before becoming a nurse, I've seen a fair amount of people dying; traumatic deaths, death from illness and death by terminal conditions; young, old and in between.

There is no one size fits all in the matter of leaving this current earth. Though there may be some similarities in the details, each is as unique as the person themselves. And the grieving that follows these life events are not cookie cutter either. Many variables can play a part in our grieving and even be different at various times in our lives.

Though this topic can be heart-wrenching at times, the short novellas in the *Passing* series are meant to provide encouragement for your walk with Christ while battling certain life events.

Each book in the series delves into different ways one might leave this current earth and offers some reassuring details made clear by God's word as well as things often experienced by others throughout the process. All are put in story form, to show that we all have a story, we are all people, with concerns and triumphs.

I hope this novella brings some peace to your heart.

Books by Tana Osborn

Until Heaven Then My Friend - Life's Journey For Your Beloved Dog

Turning Grief Into Sweet Memories

Passing - One Man's Pilgrimage Through Cancer To Heaven

Passing - One Woman's Pilgrimage Through Alzheimer's To Heaven

Passing – One Young Man's Pilgrimage Through Suicide To Heaven (Estimated availability December 2020)

Passing – A Woman's Pilgrimage Through Rebellion and Drug Overdose To Heaven (Estimated availability March 2021)

Finding Streams in the Wasteland - The Aftermath of Suicide and a Mother's Anguish (Estimated availability July 2021)

More books to come in the *Passing* series and related series.

Stay tuned @ www.tanaosborn.com/book-release-updates

Table of Contents

Chapter 1

A High Spirited Child

Many described her as a high spirited girl. She was born in an Iowa farm town in the early 1920s. She tended the horses, cows, chickens, sheep and pigs every day before going to school and again when she got home. She loved it! She didn't mind that it was hard sometimes or if she got a little manure on her clothes. The smell of the barnyard was comforting.

Her parents had to keep a close watch as sometimes they'd look over across their farm only to see Betty Jo out in the field on her horse roping a cow. If she roped the cow successfully, she would then ride up to the cow and slide off the side of her saddle-less horse onto the cow's back. She would squeeze her little legs around the sides of the cow's belly and throw her arms around their neck as far as she could reach. Sometimes the cows would buck up and down, even side to side, but sometimes they'd just run off in their effort to get this little human off their back. Though the cows were used to her and didn't get too wild, it was enough to land her on the ground a few times. Amazingly, she did often manage to stay on the cow for a fairly long time, then rather uneventfully slide off their backs.

There was one cow, who actually didn't seem to mind at all. She would just continue grazing blissfully. She wouldn't even run from the flying whoosh of the rope past her ear. These two seemed to have an odd trusting relationship.

When Betty Jo started these parent frazzling behaviors, for the first several months, her dad would run over to scold her as he was concerned for her safety. He knew his wife was at her wit's end to keep this child safe from her own antics. After a while though, it seemed pointless as this child ran her life on her terms. They'd stop her from one thing, then she'd just be onto something else. She even rode the pigs at times. That never went well and she always ended up quite hideously filthy. She also took to roping the turkeys and chickens when not on horseback. Quite the sight to see this 10-year-old little girl running around the yard roping fowl. They certainly didn't appreciate it any more than her mom and dad did. Awful nerve-wracking squaking could be heard all across the whole farmyard with the ferocious fluttering of wings and their feathers flying.

Betty Jo wasn't a bad child. She did all her chores without ever grumbling. She was helpful and polite in the home and at school, though her school work sometimes suffered as she stared outside of the one window little red schoolhouse rather than listening. Undoubtedly, thinking up new mischief. She always finished her schoolwork before either of her siblings, so she could run out and do other things. And she nearly always obeyed her parents except when it came to her farm antics. She didn't mean to be disobedient or worry her parents, but these ideas seemed to just take over and her body followed. After a while, her parents came to accept that this was just part of who Betty Jo was.

As her dad came to this reality that there was no stopping her, her dad started helping her learn more things around the farm, so she could at least know how she can do things more safely. He taught her how to ride bulls and wild horses, little ones of course; if there is any such thing as little ones when your treasured child is put on them. She reveled in this knowledge and was nearly always the first to volunteer with anything that needed to be done on the farm. She helped with fence repairing, running the plow, planting, harvesting, feeding, cleaning and birthing animals.

When Betty Jo turned 12, her dad taught her how to handle a revolver and a rifle. She was quite the marksman. She started going on hunting trips with her father. She had quite the eagle eye to spot the ring-necked pheasants in the area. She was very proud that she was able to contribute to the feeding of her family.

Chapter 2

Farm Life Turns More Difficult

Their farm had always been reasonably successful. Not much went into savings, but bills were paid and everyone was fed. Times started getting pretty difficult though in the early 1930s. Crops were not getting the prices they used to and many people were losing their farms. A lot of farmers burned their corn in their stoves to keep warm as they couldn't afford coal. It smelled like popcorn in the neighborhood sometimes. Betty Jo always loved that smell, though not the reason it smelled like that in their community.

Betty Jo and her siblings sometimes skipped school to do odd jobs around town for a little extra money, but even city dwellers were struggling and often there wasn't any odd jobs to be found. Sometimes if they could not find the wild game to feed their family, they would have to eat some of their farm animals meant to sell to others. They shared some of this with their neighbors who didn't have that option.

Though not easy, their family did get through that time and managed to keep their farm. Betty Jo grew into a very sweet, yet tough young lady. Many of the young males her age were a bit intimated by her traditionally male skills and she got her fair share of ruthless teasing. However, there were others enamored with her beautiful and kind spirit.

Chapter 3

The Start Of Something

Betty Jo eventually got the attention of William, a young man who was particularly smitten with her. He felt sad for her that she had to endure such senseless teasing, which even sometimes progressed to pushing and taunting. William began to step in and would quickly curtail any such bullying, at times to his detriment. It would not deter him, however. He loved her and was determined to protect her. This did not go unnoticed by Betty Jo. Even though she had not been too interested in being in a serious relationship with a man like so many of her friends were, her heart quickly softened to William who always treated her kindly. When he smiled at her, her heart would flutter inside her chest. She would feel all giddy inside.

As their relationship grew, the giddiness changed to something even more beautiful that there just aren't any words to describe. It became like some type of contented smile that illuminated in her soul. She thought for sure, he would propose to her and before too long, he did.

William was of an average build and a hard-working man who had lost his parents several years before meeting Betty Jo. Though he couldn't afford a farm of his own yet, he did do tenant farming, not far from Betty Jo. There had been a couple of girlfriends, but nothing serious. The interest just wasn't real strong in advancing either of those relationships. After Betty Jo came into his life, that all changed. His smile seemed to attach to his eyes as they would immediately sparkle when he smiled at Betty Jo. She noticed it, but William told her that it was her beauty that made his eyes brighten when he smiled in her direction. They spent some wonderful months together and their love for each other grew.

Chapter 4

The Bumbling Proposal

After several months of spending every spare moment together, he could not wait any longer to ask her to be his wife. He wanted to ask her father for his blessing first, but he was nervous. He had a great rapport with her father, but this was huge and he wondered if it would be enough?

One day, he mustered up the courage to speak with whom he hoped would be his father-in-law. William hid in the bushes near the barn where her father was working, waiting for the opportune time when Betty Jo was busy in her house. He wanted to speak with him privately about his desired intention.

Finally, he was alone in the barn, so he clandestinely approached. The door was ajar, so he quietly slithered into the barn. Though he was typically a courageous, self-confident man, he sheepishly shuffled over to Betty Jo's father. He felt like he was drenched in trepidation sweat.

He repeated to himself that, of course, he would give his blessing as they had developed such a good relationship over the last few months. Then doubtful thoughts would sneak in that got him thinking that maybe her father was just being nice to him or maybe he likes him okay, but maybe he didn't think he was good enough for his daughter. Then one doubtful thought after another bombarded him, even to the point of pausing his shuffle and almost turning around. Engrossed in this battle of positive and negative thoughts and scenarios, he didn't see the bucket in front of him and he stumbled over it. He started falling sideways, instinctively grabbing the rake which was leaning against the barn stall, then doing a near cartwheel landing him in the cow manure.

Betty Jo's father saw William when he came into the barn, but didn't let on. He suspected the reason he came to see him as he knew the day would be arriving soon. He could tell he was more than a bit apprehensive and he figured it was an opportunity to have a little fun. When he fell in the manure pile though, he almost lost it. Instead, he controlled his laughter, slightly glanced his way and just said, "Hey, there's a bucket there."

William fought his instinct to get up and run out the barn door from embarrassment, but instead, he got up, brushed what he could off of him, took a deep breath and moved forward.

Betty Jo's father loved William and was so grateful

for him in so many ways. Just a few months prior, if he didn't know his character enough before the storm of storms, he certainly knew it after. There was such great tragedy for Betty Jo's father related to the storm that autumn day of November 11th,1940. It seemed to surprise everyone and death came with it. Many lives were lost and It destroyed much of Iowa's horticulture and poultry.

Chapter 5

Armistice Day Blizzard Brings Tragedy

Iowa was second in the production of apple trees, but that awful blizzard in November took out a great deal of them. With the threat of war approaching, many farmers felt it was just too risky and expensive to start the process of planting more apple trees as it could take up to 5 years to get a profitable harvest.

A great many farmers turned to faster growing crops like corn and soybeans. Betty Jo's father was one of them, who chose to focus more on corn crops after that instead of apples. To make the farm devastation worse, it had also rained heavily the two days before the temperatures dropped from being 50 degrees to zero in less than 24 hours.

Some places reported a 30 degree drop in temperature in the course of two hours and snowdrifts up to 5 feet. And because of these heavy rains prior, the turkeys who had soaked feathers froze when the blizzard hit. It is now known as the Armistice Day blizzard. One that would not be forgotten.

The real pain though was not the financial blow, but personal, as he lost two of his children that day. His son, Betty Jo's brother had gone to the upper Mississippi River to join thousands of duck hunters. As this particular autumn had been unusually warm, most of the hunters packed lighter clothes. Betty Jo's father often went on this popular duck hunting day but wasn't able to go this time, but his son and his son's friend headed up to upper Mississippi River on their own. His daughter, Betty Jo's sister, went along as well to be dropped off in town as one of her friends had moved to the area and she took the opportunity to travel with her brother to visit her.

It was sunny and 55 degrees when their hunting trip began. This historic storm that had hit the pacific northwest, even taking out the Tacoma Narrows Bridge was headed their way. Though most storms coming from there usually lose their vigor while crossing the Rockies, this one didn't. It courted moisture from the Gulf of Mexico and cold air from Canada and soon walloped the region. Skies grew dark and winds and rain began. By about noon, a blizzard was firmly upon them.

At first, a lot of the hunters didn't realize the full extent of why the ducks were in large groups. They were excited and unaware that the ducks were trying to flee the approaching storm. Many stayed to get as many as possible before the 4 pm closing deadline. By then though, the blizzard was formidable and there was no easy way back to any reliable refuge. The river waves rose to 5 foot and they overwhelmed many hunters trying to reach the shore. Some tried to shelter under overturned boats or in potholes or bushes while some just tried to keep walking around in an effort to stay warm.

Betty Jo's father was told later by a neighbor who was duck hunting that he was close to them when their boat capsized shortly before reaching shore. They tried to reach each other. Though the boys were able to get hold of each other, the neighbor ended up further down the river, but was able to survive the ordeal.

The boys were able to get onto land, but their boat broke apart and was lost. At this point, the storm was so ominous, there was no way to tell which way to go through the wailing winds and pelting snow. They did their best to dig a shelter in the already increasing snow accumulation to at least decrease the wind chill, which by night time would reach 55 below zero.

Both boys were eventually found dead. They were taken to Winona, Minnesota, where there was a city garage that was being used as a temporary morgue for the frozen hunters recovered. Many of the men brought there were so frozen, bodies had to thaw before an identification could be searched for. Many of the hunters there were from out of town.

Betty Jo's sister had been in town with her friend weathering things out but was stricken with such worry as she hadn't heard from her brother since the storm hit. The news did come back from some of those who had gone out to rescue people that there were many casualties to the weather. She was eventually told that some of those found frozen were being taken to Winona.

Though it took days to clear some of the roads, she did find someone who her friend knew that was headed in that direction. He was willing to take her along. Her and the driver of the car were found later over an embankment. He was barely alive, but she did not fare even that well.

Word did get back to Betty Jo and of course, her mother and father that their son and daughter had died. This was the most emotionally distressing time in all their lives. William was heartbroken for all of them. It was hard to know even what to say. Not having any words that could take their sadness away, he showed his compassion and empathy by helping as much as he could around their farm.

William helped with disposing of the turkeys that had froze due to the rain before the storm getting their feathers so wet, then causing them to freeze in the storm. He also repaired a great deal of the barn damage. He worked on helping the apple trees recover, at least the ones that looked like they could be saved. He was also instrumental in his assistance in keeping the morale up in their family and comforting Betty Jo. It could never be enough to heal their hearts from such a tragedy, but it was all he had to give.

Betty Jo's father knew William was a man of great caliber before this, but he was convinced of it after seeing how tirelessly he worked to make sure they were safe, physically, emotionally and financially. He could not have picked a better man to marry his daughter. And in the wake of his son and daughter's absence, he was even more appreciative of William.

Chapter 6

Continuation Of The Proposal

Betty Jo's father was enjoying William's nervousness and he watched out the corner of his eye as William picked himself up off the barn floor, brushing the dirt off his trousers with his head down. He tried with all his might not to laugh at the predicament William had created for himself.

After William got up, he took two quick steps toward Betty Jo's father and quickly blurted out, "Sir, I love Betty Jo and I want to spend all my days providing and protecting her," he paused, lovingly lowered his voice and slowly said, "and just loving her, Sir. Would we have your blessing?"

Betty Jo's father had hoped to make William sweat a bit more, but he was overwhelmed with joy and felt bad for his mishap, so the best he could do was to matter-of-factly say to William, "Well, you kind of smell like manure."

There was an awkward pause in the interaction, but it didn't last long as he could not contain his happiness that William wanted to marry Betty Jo. He threw his arms around him despite the cow manure that still was on William's clothes and reassured William that he had his blessing and reassured him that he knew Betty Jo's mother would be thrilled as well.

William thanked him and reassured him that he would take good care of his daughter. He did ask William to set the wedding date at least after she was 18 though, which he agreed, as it was only a couple of months away.

Chapter 7

William And Betty Jo Married

A couple of months later William and Betty Jo got married on her father's farm. It was a joyous day for all. As a wedding gift, her father gave them 10 acres of his farmland in which they could start their life together. It was a wonderful part of his land that he just hadn't got around to cultivating. It even had a small creek that went along part of it.

It wasn't long after they finished building their farmhouse that William was drafted into World War II in April of 1943. Their souls were heavy with the thought of being separated.

There was some concern that Betty Jo's father would be drafted as well with the draft age extended for people in their 40's, but he was not. If he had, it would have been devastating for both of their farms. As it was, he, his wife and Betty Jo worked both farms to the point of utter exhaustion at times in order to keep up with things.

Betty Jo loved farm work just like she did when she

was a child. Her dad loved watching Betty Jo interacting with the animals or even work out in the fields because she was always smiling. Even when totally exhausted, she just didn't seem to mind.

Soon after William left for war, it was discovered that she was pregnant. She was so excited, but also sad because William was not there with her. Her parents stepped in to reassure her and offered to take over chores if she needed to rest.

Betty Jo was a tough young woman though who typically did not let anything keep her down. When her morning sickness lasted for hours every morning and kept her from successfully keeping any food in her stomach, she still insisted on doing her farm chores. Her parents just smiled and shook their heads as they watched her go from chore to chore carrying her vomit bucket with her.

Her father had given her and William the cow, who as a child would just let Betty Jo sit on her back while grazing, now almost 20. The cow just watched Betty Jo and would "moo" any time Betty Jo used her bucket. When she and the cow were close, the cow sniffed at her like she knew she was pregnant or maybe that she was feeling ill. Betty Jo's father had been around cows all his life and he knew that they can be quite intuitive creatures in sensing what is going on in our human emotions, but he had never seen a cow so connected as this one was to Betty Jo.

Betty Jo wanted to do her share, but her parents did help to lighten the load as best they could while still keeping their own farm going. The morning sickness did improve and Betty Jo felt comfortable working her farm and helping her parents. Her and her mom planned great meals in order to keep up everyone's health and energy the best they could.

Betty Jo worked up to the birth of her daughter, only redistributed some of the tasks that were not safe to her father. Farm work did slow down though as she approached her 8th month in November. Her daughter Willa was born in December, right on time. Betty Jo's mother was there helping her get through the contractions of her labor. She was fortunate that though there was snow on the ground, it was a clear day and an easy jaunt for the doctor and midwife to come to see her. Willa came out healthy, but protesting the journey to her new world. She quieted down as soon as she was placed in her mother's arms.

Betty Jo beamed with joy and sadness at the same time. She so wished William was there with her, but this little girl distracted her from that yearning in her heart. In the first few weeks of taking care of little Willa, she could barely focus on anything except just surviving between the lack of sleep and relentless crying.

After a few weeks though, Willa was doing better with sleeping and this helped Betty Jo regain a little more alertness. She had heard back from William, who appeared quite ecstatic about him becoming a father.

She could tell from the writing of his letter that he was weepy when writing it. He knew he would not likely be back with Betty Jo for a while yet and was saddened thinking about all he was missing, but he knew he couldn't change that right now and needed to focus on his tasks at war for now.

It was difficult raising Willa without William around, but her parents helped tremendously. When that first spring came and it was time to get the fields ready for planting, Betty Jo put her baby in a pack and got to it. Her dad did the heavy machine work.

As the season came and went, William still was not back and by Christmas, Willa was taking a few wobbly steps. Betty Jo tried to keep William up to date on all that was going on at home and that they were okay. When William was able, he wrote back.

When the following spring came, Willa was old enough to understand a little about what goes on at the farm, but certainly didn't appreciate the dangers, so Betty Jo kept a tight watch on her. Betty Jo struggled a bit with depression, but never let onto her parents and certainly not her daughter. She missed William. There were a few people in town who thought the war would be ending soon. Soon was not soon enough for Betty Jo. There were many nights, she literally cried herself to sleep as she ached so deeply for William.

Chapter 8

William Returns From War

Finally, in September of 1945, the war ended. William returned thinner and noticeably weary in appearance, but the sight of Betty Jo made all that he had experienced in war vanish instantly, at least for that moment. They embraced with a myriad of tears flowing between them. The last 29 months seemed like an eternity to both of them.

Watching from an open door to their little farmhouse were two little eyes, wondering if this could be her father who her mommy had talked about. Betty Jo directed William's eyes to those watching him so intently from the open door. He stood, almost puzzled looking for a moment, then another torrent of tears began to fall from his eyes as it sunk in that this was his daughter.

This little girl, conceived shortly before he left for war was now a toddler. She locked eyes with her daddy and ran as fast as her little new walking legs would move to say hello. Daddy swooped her up in his arms and embraced his daughter with another bout of tears streaming down his face.

As the weeks unfolded after William's return, it became apparent that he was suffering from some troubling memories of the things he experienced in war. He'd toss and turn, mumbling, sometimes striking out in his sleep. Oftentimes, he'd start that way then abruptly sit up and yell out, which would wake up all in the house. A look of fright, sometimes anger was all over his face. Betty Jo learned to wait a few moments before trying to reassure him. At first, she would grab his hand to comfort him, but those first few moments he was still on the battlefield in his mind and he would jerk away and by reflex start to strike out. Betty Jo learned to duck very quickly and let go of his hand.

They were told that William was experiencing CSR or Combat Stress Reaction or "battle fatigue." He was able to function pretty well in the daytime as he was busy with farm and ranch chores. Even after he came in, he was absorbed by his wonderful daughter and Betty Jo. It was his favorite part of the day. Even when things got quieter after little Willa went to bed, William was fine sitting by the fireplace with Betty Jo, whether talking or not. It was when he laid down at bedtime with no other distractions that war memories would try to sneak into his thoughts.

He worked hard at trying to redirect those thoughts

to something much more positive. He was sometimes successful, sometimes not. And after asleep, it was out of his control. Some nights were fine, others not.

There were times Betty Jo just didn't know if he would ever work through those horrible memories. She wondered if she was doing enough to help. She tried to always be supportive, but she felt very limited in what she could do. She could be there for him, but he had to work through it on his own timing. He did see the doctor every now and then. They talked about things a bit. The town doctor had seen a fair amount of other men who had returned from war with similar symptoms.

William never wanted to tell Betty Jo any details as he was always trying to protect her. He knew his difficulties with this Combat Stress Reaction would only trouble her and he felt awful for making her worry as it is. He did feel so blessed to have her by his side though. She often thought it might help if he would talk to her more about it, but he never did.

Eventually, the nightmares did become less and less. Though flashbacks did occur from time to time, William was able to handle them more effectively and they were less intense. He was so thankful for the patience his dear wife had for him as he worked through these troubling flashbacks.

Life pretty much went on with the typical ups and

downs, joys and challenges with life and of course, raising little Willa. William and Betty Jo had a few disagreements here and there, but they were always able to talk them out, sooner or later. They were always looking out for each other and this kept them going strong.

Willa loved the farm life just like her mother did. She loved taking care of the animals and helping with all the farm chores when she wasn't at school. She wasn't quite as wild as her mother was growing up, but just as helpful to her parents.

Chapter 9

The Tractor Tragedy

There were many changes throughout the years with the ways of transportation and machines to assist with farming and ranching. With the improved technology, it made their work quite a bit easier. Some of the machinery was dangerous though. The tractors caused many injuries as they rolled over easily and crushed farmers. They did become safer when they began making them with rollover protective structures and seat-belts, but those weren't standard until the 80's in the United States.

The timing of those safety improvements did not help Betty Jo's mother that blustery slimy muddy day in autumn when she was riding the tractor. Betty Jo's father was ill with the flu and so achy and congested, he couldn't even get out of bed without help. He typically worked the farm no matter how rotten he felt, but this was different. He had been generally quite healthy and robust, even in his sixties. This bug though had knocked him flat.

Willa was off at college, so wasn't able to help out

on the farm. William knew that his father-in-law had not been feeling well, so he had been coming over every morning to see if he needed help with anything. Betty Jo's mother figured William would be over soon, but that she would get started, so she could harvest some corn while still cool outside.

They often harvested their corn early in the morning as it was easier to get the heat out of the corn and prevent it from going into starch, but with him being ill, they weren't able to do that. She got out as soon as she had her husband taken care of and resting. The sun wasn't quite up yet, so it was still dim when she was able to get outside.

It had rained pretty heavily that morning and actually was still drizzling. The ground was slick. She had helped with the farm for years and driven the tractor. Today though, as she was turning around toward the tractor attachment, her tire un-expectantly slipped in an unseen rut and the tractor rolled. In that split second when she felt the tractor rolling, she tried to correct, but it was to no avail. Tragically, the tractor rolled and stopped leaving Betty Jo's mother underneath it.

She could not yell as the weight of the tractor on her chest would not allow it and nobody was around to hear her anyway. Breathing tiny shallow breaths, diminishing a little more at each miniscule breath. She knew her life on this current earth was coming to an end.

It was like all of her life played before her in those few moments. Though not without sadness, she was so grateful for the many blessings in her life. She wanted to write in the dirt with her finger, "I love you," but she didn't have the strength. She managed to use her two fingers and made a little heart, not knowing if anyone would see it. A few moments later, she took the last breath that she could manage.

It was about an hour later, William came over to check on his in-laws. The sun was starting to shine onto their farm. As he was almost there he could see, what he thought, was unusual lighting at the edge of their farm. He felt oddly urged to investigate how the sun that was trying to peak around the clouds was actually hitting this part of their farm at this time of the morning.

To get to it, he had to go a little off the path and out of his way. As he was getting closer, he gazed intently at the unusual lighting, then he noticed the tractor rolled over and his heart sank as he then saw his mother-in-law on the ground underneath. He rushed over but found only her lifeless body remained. He slumped over her and wept.

As William slightly lifted his gaze, he took her hand, cupping it in his, he softly muttered, "I'm so sorry." As he was holding her hand close to him, it was as if that weird light was shining on some small scribble in the dirt where her hand had been. Though someone passing by would likely never have noticed such an insignificant indentation in the mud, he recognized it as a small heart. William sadly smiled and whispered, "We love you."

He found some cut logs near the barn and he wedged them under both ends of the tractor, then he dug underneath her and was able to pull her out from under the tractor. He lifted her, bringing her into the house and laying her onto the couch. He used their phone to call his friend at the police station to let him know what happened.

How was he going to tell Betty Jo's father? He made that arduous journey up the stairs to tell him what had happened. When he arrived, he found him asleep. So he decided to go tell Betty Jo first, then come back to care for his father-in-law.

It seemed like it took forever to get to his farm, just a few acres away, yet also like just a few seconds and not nearly long enough. He got home to find Betty Jo working in the kitchen. She saw his pensive expression and knew something was wrong. William gently took her hand and brought her to sit down at the kitchen table. She sat in a locked gaze, trying to absorb the news, then after a pause, tears began to fall and William moved his chair closer. She buried her face into his chest. They sat together like this for several minutes. She then lifted her head and asked, "How is Dad?"

William explained that he was asleep and he hadn't told him yet. He had always worked through illnesses before. They were wondering if he had gotten worse from yesterday and whether that was why her mom was trying to work on the farm for him. Betty Jo and William decided to assess how he was doing and whether he could deal with such a tragic revelation.

Chapter 10

Telling Her Father

William and Betty Jo went back to see her father. He was awake but appeared weak. He could barely hold the water cup. Betty Jo made some soup for him and he ate a little bit with her help. He did have a low-grade fever. They felt it was time to call the doctor even though her father had resisted that notion prior.

The doctor was able to come out that day and told them he likely had a very bad case of influenza, which is trying to settle into pneumonia. He gave him some antibiotics and instructed them to help him get plenty of fluids. They both decided that hearing the news about his wife right now could be detrimental to his recovery. They decided to wait until he had a couple of days of antibiotics in him and hopefully feeling a little better.

William and Betty Jo spent the nights in his room and William did farm work during the day, both on his farm and his father-in-law. They sufficiently distracted him from really grasping that his wife wasn't with him.

In a couple of days, he was feeling a little bit better.

He was able to eat and drink more on his own. He was able to walk himself safely and steadily to the bathroom. He had regained some of his strength. It was obvious that he had turned the corner on his illness.

William and Betty Jo felt it was time to tell him what had happened. He was starting to ask where his wife was and getting worried. They could not put it off any longer. Betty Jo sat on the side of the bed next to her dad. She began by saying, "please forgive us, Dad, for waiting a couple of days to tell you this. You were very sick and we did not feel that you could safely process the information." She proceeded to tell him how mom had gone out to help with farm chores and getting some of the corn harvested while it was cool outside. He listened in a shock-like trance. His facial expression seemed to fade into a distant withdrawal, then without saying a word, he turned over, away from Betty Jo, closed his eyes and only the faintness of his respiration was heard.

Betty Jo looked at her dad, then at William, then back at her dad. She didn't know what to say. "Dad?" She gently put her arm on his shoulder, but he said nothing. William motioned for her to leave the bedside, "I think he needs time to process all this." Betty Jo told her dad that she would let him rest now, but if he wanted to talk, she would be there for him.

All this time, William's feelings of guilt smoldered inside. He was blaming himself for not coming to their farm earlier. Maybe he could have prevented this. Though typically quite even-tempered, he began to act with brusque responses to simple interactions with Betty Jo. She didn't know what was going on but knew it was not like William. She suspected though that he felt responsible for her mother's death. She tried to take his hand and as he pulled it away briskly, she blurted out to him, "William, this is not your fault!" Her generally self-controlled husband instantly exploded in sobs and a plethora of apologies for not being at the farm earlier. Betty Jo worked feverishly to tell him that he had no way of knowing her mom would decide to go out early and not wait for him or to even anticipate this accident. It slowed the sobs of regret, but she knew she would have to reinforce this, likely many times.

Chapter 11

He Visits The Site

As they were discussing these things on the couch, they heard a voice calling from up the stairs, "Betty Jo!" Betty Jo darted to his room immediately and William behind her. When they got to his room, her father was sitting on the edge of the bed, fully dressed. "Will you take me to where this happened?" William and Betty Jo got on either side of him and steadied him as they went down the stairs and outside to where the accident occurred.

William explained that he and some friends had already set the tractor back upright and put it back in the barn the day after it happened, but William brought him to the spot. He explained that it was very muddy and slick that morning and in fact, was still drizzling when he found her. He explained that there was a rut in the mud where it appeared the tractor tire caught on, though he had filled it in after they had removed the tractor.

Betty Jo's father knelt down and slowly stroked the dirt where his wife had been. His hand paused in the dirt, his eyes closed and he was silent for a while as if he was spending those last moments together. Tears were creeping out the side of his closed eyelids, then he stood up, sighed and briskly wiped the tears away.

William had forgotten in all that had gone on since the accident that he had used his mother-in-law's Polaroid camera from the house to take a photo of the heart she fingered in the dirt. He had placed it on the bookshelf. When his father-in-law stood up, William spoke, "Dad, I want to show you and Betty Jo something," and he led them to the bookshelf in the house, "I found this fingered in the dirt," he told them, as he showed them the photo.

Betty Jo stared at the photo intently as tears meandered from her eyes down her cheeks. She then wrapped her arms around William and he held her with the reassuring embrace she so desperately needed. Her father took the photo, brought it into his chest and went to sit down on the couch.

Betty Jo walked to the kitchen to make some tea for everyone. William walked over to her father and sat down beside him. "Sir, I am so sorry that I did not get here sooner that morning to prevent this from happening." Without looking up, he replied to William, "son, this was not your fault." And no more was spoken.

Chapter 12

The Years Rolled Onto This

The next several years were fairly uneventful other than Betty Jo's father passing away a few years after his wife. Their daughter finished college and took a job about 500 miles from them. They saw her mostly on holidays.

William and Betty Jo were always looking out for each other, more concerned about the other's needs than their own. They had a special bond. There was an occasional disagreement, but they always managed to work things out and their love and respect for each other never wavered. They had something very special.

Shortly after Betty Jo's 65th birthday, William started noticing that Betty Jo frequently would forget things and wasn't retaining information as well as she used to. At first, it was subtle and he didn't think much of it, but then it became more apparent. Betty Jo was noticing it too and at first, made jokes about it. It didn't seem to affect her much on the surface. She could still socialize, although sometimes she needed a reminder about the rules of her favorite card games. She also might occasionally have trouble finding the right word for things in her conversations.

One of her most favorite places continued to be out in the farmyard, watching the cows or horses run around. And she still loved doing barnyard chores. It still made her feel comfortable and loved, just like it did when she was a youngster.

Betty Jo didn't bring up her growing concerns to William, but her forgetting things was beginning to cause her anxiety. She first attributed them to just getting older, although she didn't feel that old yet physically. William was always looking out for ways to help her without her realizing he was doing so. He knew but was afraid to mention it to her.

After a couple of years or so, things began to get worse. William started noticing that Betty Jo was not wanting to meet with friends anymore. She preferred to just stay at home and didn't do well with changes. If she did go to the market or meet a friend, she often would say something snippy and walk away. She was having an increasingly difficult time processing information and this was worse when outside her familiar environment. She frequently had to ask William about what day it was and even the time. In the morning, she'd often stare in her closet not knowing what to put on for the day.

There was no doubt now that something was definitely wrong. One evening when they were cuddled up on the couch with the relaxing glow of the fireplace, William decided to voice his concern. "Betty Jo, I've been noticing that you get upset easy lately and are having some trouble understanding conversations."

She did not say a word, but quickly buried her face into his chest and sobbed. He held her snug against him with his reassuring embrace she had come to so appreciate. After a while, he told her that he'd like for her to go to the doctor. Not moving her face out of his chest, she nodded.

Chapter 13

The Doctor Delivers The Devastating News

The next day they went to their town doctor. He did many tests and listened to all of the things they had been noticing over the last couple of years. He did many cognitive exercises with her also. He left the room for quite a while, then returned with some pamphlets about Alzheimer's.

Alzheimer's had been becoming a more recognized disease in the eighties. From what was being described, he told them she appeared to be in transition from early to mid-stage. He told them everyone is a little different, but many people in mid-stage can be in that stage for several years and others can move through quickly. The doctor explained some things to watch for and ways to help get through those challenges.

The news was devastating. Their spirits sunk. Neither spoke the whole way home. What could either of them say? They were having an agonizing time even letting it all sink in and just what it all meant and would mean for their future.

Chapter 14

A Treasured Moment Amid The Worry

The sun was brightly shining in the window the next morning. Betty Jo lay quietly on her bed. William had gotten up to make some breakfast. He didn't sleep too well. He wondered what he was going to do to keep her safe and happy. He wanted so desperately to just take all this away from her, but he knew they had to just walk through it together, moment by moment. He pondered during the sleepless night a great many things. It was a sad disease and so difficult for him to watch his sweet wife go through it. He agonized at the thought it would get worse. There were moments he cherished though.

Even that morning when he brought her breakfast while she was still in bed. He brought her some orange juice, eggs and toast just as she began to rustle in the blankets. He placed it on the bedside tray. She saw him coming with it and sat up with appreciation. He snuggled the tray against her. "Hi dear, would you like some breakfast?" She gazed at the tray and the food upon it. She paused briefly then without further hesitation, took hold of her orange juice glass and began to pour some onto her toast. William began to formulate words and lurch forward to stop her, but curtailed that response. It didn't matter and would only serve to potentially upset her, making her sad or angry. Who was he to tell her that she couldn't put orange juice on her toast? Maybe she'd like it.

It was sad that her thought process couldn't distinguish her breakfast, but it was also a treasured moment for William because as she began eating her orange juice toast, she made sweet comments to him about how yummy the pancake was and that she had never had one so good. William smiled and sat down next to her while she ate. She got a toast bite on her fork, rubbed it in the orange juice and motioned for William to have a bite, which he cautiously did. He was surprised that it actually wasn't bad that way. He learned as things progressed that it usually was better to just go along with these harmless moments of confusion than to point out she was "doing it wrong," as that would only make her sad or cause her to be upset in some way.

For a while, these little moments of poor thought process were off and on, some being minor and at times, worse. There were gaps in between that she seemed without much noticeable deficit. William adapted their lifestyle a bit to make sure she was happy and safe. Sometimes she'd come with him when working on the farm. He had made several covered comfortable sitting areas where she could watch him work and he could check on her frequently. She seemed happiest when she could watch him work or help him with the animals. Farm chores and animals had always brought her the most peace. She seemed content to watch most of the time, but at times, she tried to help as this had always been a big part of her life. It was not easy for her to understand why William just wanted her to watch him. She got upset at him sometimes for not letting her help. He was able to explain it to her, though it took a repeated effort, that she was helping him by just watching from the special places he made for her. When she latched on that she was helping him by doing what he asked, she was surprisingly content to watch most of the time.

Things sort of stabilized for the most part at the early to mid-stage range for just over a year with only an occasional mishap. Then symptoms started the dreaded progression through mid-stage and beyond.

Chapter 15

Progressing Symptoms

Betty Jo's ability to think things through and remember continued to deteriorate. William sometimes felt like she wasn't even the woman he once knew anymore. She was often withdrawn, restless at night and needing more help with daily tasks. He now had to help her every day to pick out appropriate clothes for the weather and remind her to shower. Sometimes, she would be quite amenable to these suggestions, but at other times, it would make her get frustrated and angry.

William often pushed back the feelings that Betty Jo had already left him. He grieved for the wife he once knew before the Alzheimer's took her away. He had to remind himself that the woman he loved was, in fact, still there. Her spirit, the essence of who she was, hadn't changed. It was just the illness that had damaged brain tissue that would not allow her spirit to express itself in the same way that she normally would.

He faithfully listened to her repeat things over and over and was patient with her when she got irritated because he didn't understand what she wanted. Though

53

he felt strongly that it was a gift to be able to care for his wife as she progressed through this disease, it was not always easy. He wondered if he was doing enough for her. There were days that he had many doubts that he could provide all she needed from him.

He did get some help, during the day on occasion, so he could do the needed farm and maintenance on the farm or go shopping. A lot of times, she would still come out with him and watch him work, but other times, she didn't want to leave the house. It was getting more difficult as she often could not keep her attention with him and would start to wander. He worried she might leave the house and he wouldn't know. There were times when he had to neglect some chores as he didn't feel comfortable leaving her alone at home.

Chapter 16

Concern For Safety

He had tried to allow her to be home alone, but he quickly realized her confusion had escalated when she walked off one day. She was nowhere to be found when he returned from working in the barn. That day was one of the scariest days of his life. He searched every room of the house frantically, looking in closets and under beds. While he was doing that, he began to smell something burning. His thoughts raced as he tried to isolate the smell, then he jolted off to the kitchen where he found her shoes in the oven with the oven turned on. They had not caught fire yet but they were starting to smoke a little, so he figured she could not have been gone for too long. He called his nearest neighbor and asked him if he had seen her, but he had not. He asked that he please call everyone he knew in the area. He then grabbed his flashlight and a coat for her and began looking outside.

There was a creek about a half-mile from their house. It was one of her favorite places. He decided to check there first. He walked at a brisk pace, trying not to fall in the dark on the uneven trail. He yelled her name over and over, "Betty Jo! Betty Jo! Please Betty Jo, where are you?"

He got to the edge of the creek. He called again, looking up and down the water's edge with his flashlight. He didn't see her. He shined the light onto the muddy ground to look for any evidence of footprints, but he didn't notice anything that would lead him to believe she had gone into the creek. Then a small glimpse of hope caught his glance. A little deepening in the dirt and a few leaves on the ground that looked like maybe the bush next to the trail might have been brushed. He moved in that direction, shining his light up ahead on the trail. He saw what looked to be a leg. "Betty Jo!"

He ran over there to find Betty Jo curled up, leaning against the side of a large rock, sleeping. He shook her, gently, but with a sort of frightened fervor. "Betty Jo?" She raised her head and smiled. She kissed his cheek and buried her face into his chest as he wrapped his arms around her. He sobbed, so grateful that she was okay. He helped her up and put the coat around her. She was barefoot. It would be too hard for her to walk with his big shoes, but he took them off, removed his socks and put his socks on her feet to protect them. Then he tore some strips off his undershirt and tied them around the upper end of the sock to help keep them from slipping down off her legs. She looked down at her "new shoes" and giggled softly.

They walked slowly back to the house, talking and laughing. Well, she was laughing. He was still trying to settle himself down from the gut-wrenching stress that was frantically coursing throughout every cell in his body surrounding the whole event.

They finally returned to the house safely. He called his neighbor to let him know he found her. William made her some warm soup, but Betty Jo got agitated when he tried to sit her at the table. He offered her some water, but she declined. He thought she must be tired and he assisted her to bed. When she saw it, she crawled in and immediately curled up in the fetal position. William tenderly pulled the blankets up over her and tucked her in. She fell asleep almost immediately.

William sat in the wooden chair kept in the bedroom and gazed upon his wife in a sad prolonged stare. Then he exhaled a long breath and with a lovingly, but bittersweet grin, he thought about how she reacted when he found her. How she gazed up at him and buried her face in his chest as she has always liked to do. The look she had on her face made him feel like he was her hero. He didn't know if she truly knew exactly who he was, but she seemed to recognize him as someone safe and familiar. He was so thankful for that and treasured that moment.

As he continued to gaze at his precious wife, a small tear made its way out of the corner of each of his eyes. He exhaustively wiped them away as he pondered about what he was going to do. He knew he could no longer leave her alone in the house.

Chapter 17
William Changes Careers

He knew at least a couple of his neighbors would be willing to be with her during the day sometimes while he worked on the farm, but this was not a long term solution. Selling the farm was not a good option as farms were in crisis at this time. He had been slowly downsizing his farm over the last few years and had been receiving social security checks. He had managed to save a little here and there and did own the farm, so he felt fairly comfortable that he could officially retire and be okay. He didn't have the money for professional nursing care, but as long as he could keep her safe, he wanted to take care of her at home anyway. After speaking with the folks at the Alzheimer's Association, a relatively new resource, he was given some idea of what he might expect in caring for her at home.

William spoke to one of his neighbors who was likely going to lose his farm and offered what harvest was forthcoming from his farm if he was able to work and care for the crops. His neighbor agreed and was very grateful for the opportunity for extra income. Then just like that, William changed professions from farmer to caregiver. The most challenging endeavor he would ever take on, yet the greatest honor for him to be able to accompany his cherished wife on this often turbulent pilgrimage through Alzheimer's disease.

Chapter 18
What About Heaven?

As Betty Jo's disease got worse to the point of her not being able to even remember him sometimes, William wondered about her salvation. She knew her Lord and Savior before this disease, but now, she often couldn't even remember her name. He asked the pastor to come to talk with him.

William thanked Pastor Steven for coming to see him, then explained to him that the Alzheimer's Association and her doctor had helped him to understand that the disease is damaging brain function and altering the patterns stored in her brain, which is causing the problems with her memory and difficulty in communicating. William expressed his lack of understanding in what it meant to her salvation as she is not capable of having a relationship with her Savior.

The pastor explained to William that she is in God's care. He reminded him of a verse in God's word, Romans 8:37-39 says "No, in all these things we are more than conquerors through him who loved us. For I am convinced that neither death nor life, neither angels nor demons, neither the present nor the future, nor any powers, neither height nor depth, nor anything else in all creation, will be able to separate us from the love of God that is in Christ Jesus our Lord."

Pastor Steven continued, "though her physical brain is being damaged by the disease, which is causing disconnect for her soul and spirit to express herself like she once did or to understand who her Savior is, her soul is still the Betty Jo you have always loved. I don't know all the facets of how this disease alters the brain, but I do know that God is in control and He will restore her completely. He doesn't turn his back on us when we suffer from physical or mental challenges."

William was encouraged but wanted more, so the pastor continued. He quoted Genesis 2:7, "And the LORD God formed man of the dust of the ground, and breathed into his nostrils the breath of life; and man became a living soul." (Quoting from the King James Version), but added, that the New International Version stated it, "… and the man became a living being."

He told him that he feels this passage indicates that the breath of life activates, if you will, our living being or soul.

He expounded on this, "This 'breath of life' is delivered to all our body cells via our blood. Without it, there is no life. It is like the fuel that moves your car from point A to point B and back to A. If you don't have gas in your car, it won't go. Similarly, your body won't function without the 'breath of life,' which makes the body a living soul or living being. In essence, it "turns you on" or gives you life, making you a living soul.

Having this breath of life brings life to our 'mind,'

which can reason, make decisions and experience emotions. Your mind is more than your brain. Your brain has incredible components that provide the opportunity to do these things, but like a computer, if you don't turn the switch on, the components are unused. We are born with the parts, but these "come alive" when we become a living being.

Betty Jo's brain components though are damaged, so even though the switch is in the on position, her soul, the components are damaged so the communications or lack thereof, are being expressed chaotically. Her will, memories and decision making are part of her soul that partly have been imprinted on her brain making her who she is, but with the brain components damaged, she can't decipher a great many things anymore. Betty Jo, based on her reactions to her past experiences and thoughts have shaped who she is deep in her soul. This is what makes each treasured soul different.

Explaining someone's spirit is a bit complex. Most Bible scholars explain our spirit as the essence of who we are as a person. It is the reflection of our body and soul. It can be thought of in light of the Holy Spirit which is the essence of who God is. Our spirit is the essence of who we are. It is the deepest, most innermost part of you and is eternal.

The Bible tells us that when our body dies, our spirit (a reflection of our body and soul) will return to the God who gave it. When Jesus himself died on the cross

He said in a loud voice, "Father, into your hands I commit My spirit." When He had said this, He breathed His last. (Luke 23:46).

Your soul or mind can reason and make decisions, but it is your spirit that shapes those responses and emotions. It is your spirit that directs your life response to the physical stimuli taken in by your body senses and thoughts that come into your soul or mind because it is the innermost you, the essence of who you are.

Another way to think about it is that our spirit is like an electrical outlet that allows the connection of the Holy Spirit if we accept the gift of salvation from Jesus dying on the cross for us. When we do that we are "born again." The Holy Spirit of God plugs into our spirit, if you will, and much of our decision making and thought process will involve His influence.

Though Betty Jo may not understand all this right now due to the damage being done in her brain connections, God is plugged into her spirit and when her body dies, her spirit will return to Him.

The Bible tells us that if there is a natural body, there is also a spiritual body and it will be raised. That's your spirit, a reflection of your body and soul," Pastor Steven explained.

William pondered all this. He began to understand, somewhat anyway, but that he need not worry about the salvation of his wife and that her spirit was alive and well. She just wasn't able to express herself as she once did due to the damage being done to her brain patterns and connections from Alzheimer's.

Of course, she couldn't reason all this out as he could. It made him think just how confusing and scary it must be for her. He renewed his determination to try to make these last days of her life as pleasant as they could be as they both made this pilgrimage through Alzheimer's together.

Chapter 19
Holding Onto The Good

The daily road through her Alzheimer's was a bit rocky at times. One common part of her day could go the same predictable way for days at a time, then all a sudden, the same particular task could make her very upset. It left William wondering what part went wrong, but it wasn't the activity as much as just how she was processing things at that moment. She got to the point also where her perception of pain was altered. She couldn't express that she had pain or even if she was uncomfortable in some other way. William tried hard to determine if her behavior might be related to pain sometimes. He sharpened his observation skills in what her body language might be telling him, especially her facial expressions or tensions which might be tight or grimacing. This would at least tell him to try to make her more comfortable.

Depending on what non-verbal signs she might be showing him, he might try to give her a shoulder rub or take a little walk with her. He would give her some Tylenol if nothing else was helping. She didn't always cooperate with taking her medications though. She also had a daily blood pressure pill, but either of them was hit and miss. If he even dare to crush them and put them in applesauce, who knows if she would be amenable or

67

not. She could take them, but just as easily spit them out at him.

For a while, sitting outside with her while she watched the farm animals was her favorite calming activity. As things progressed though, she wouldn't sit still very long and tended to want to wander. It was difficult to get her to come back in, so William didn't do it anymore. He didn't have many left, as he had gotten rid of most of his farm animals when he chose to retire from farming, so it would free up more time for Betty Jo.

Their life wasn't easy, but he reminded himself daily and on the more challenging days, several times a day, that Betty Jo had no way of expressing herself as she used to because of the damaged disconnections in her brain. It was his job to help her navigate and he devoted himself to this task. There were times when he felt so drained that he just couldn't do it anymore and would reach out for help from his daughter or friends. He did feel a bit guilty for those times, even though he knew caregiver stress was a natural part of taking care of his wife 24/7 and that it didn't mean he didn't love his wife. Still, he just wanted to make her life as good as it could be. He soon recognized that when he felt this way, asking a friend to come sit with her for even an hour or two was the best thing he could do for her.

His daughter, Willa, was able to come out for a few days every couple of months. This was when he would often go somewhere to recharge. Willa had a harder time though in helping Betty Jo as she hadn't spent a lot of time with her mother for many years as she lived so far away. Betty Jo only rarely recognized her. Willa's explanation that she was her daughter helped Betty Jo engage sometimes, but that became less and less as she progressed.

William drew strength for the patience he needed and challenges he faced from the generally sweet times they had together. It was a lot of work, helping her with all the tasks of daily living like dressing, bathing, feeding and the like, but he usually did well getting her through the tasks a good part of the day.

Betty Jo did have difficult times of confusion and anxiety sometimes though. The most difficult times for William were when she accused him of stealing something or the times she was afraid as she didn't know who he was. These were some of the worse moments of his life. He would repeatedly remind himself that it was the disease, but it was heart-wrenching as it just reinforced how his precious wife's memories were gone. To see his confident, sweet, nearly fearless wife be so anxious was unbearable. He did his best to console her during these times and get her through, but it was not an easy task. He often later would withdraw and weep for her. Fortunately, they only occurred on occasion.

When she did get exceptionally confused about who he was, she would often try to leave. He quickly learned that he had to install deadbolts and hide the keys, so she would not run out the doors and get lost.

One day, before he realized she would exit, she got

scared and ran out the door. William was right there with her, but he wasn't able to stop her before she managed to get outside and head purposefully toward the road. Talking to her or offering to walk with her only made her walk faster. He had to stealthily follow her until she calmed down. That day, he walked at least a mile before he could see that she was walking calmly. When she started pausing and looking around like she was trying to figure out where she was, he re-approached her. He tested the waters first, just saying a friendly hello, then commenting on the weather. Then he said, "Betty Jo, are you headed back home? You mind if I walk with you?" Her face had shown that she wasn't sure how to get back home and was appearing a bit weary, so when he said that, he believed somewhere in her, she knew the way back home was with him. After that event, William put deadbolts on the doors and hoped she wouldn't try to get out the windows. The windows had never been easy to open, so he felt comfortable she could not open them.

Chapter 20
The Reassuring Embrace

What William treasured most about this pilgrimage through Alzheimer's, and there certainly wasn't a lot to treasure, was the comfort she still often received from his embrace. Before her disease, she had always burrowed her face into his chest when she was upset or needed reassurance and he would wrap his arms around her and hold her. She once told him that it was like getting an infusion of peace when she was feeling disharmony or unrest in her spirit. With her battle with Alzheimer's, she wouldn't always let him hold her for this infusion of sorts, but this embrace still was the one constant that she latched onto when she was confused or even agitated. Sometimes he would offer to hold her, but often she would grab hold of him as she had always done, then nuzzle her face into his chest while he held her. In the helplessness to make his wife be happier, William felt so blessed that he could still offer comfort to Betty Jo in this small way.

There was one time when she was crying and yelling at him, though he had no clue why. He tried to give her Tylenol thinking maybe she was uncomfortable, but she threw it at him. He tried to offer her some water and a snack, but one swoop of her hand sent it flying off the table. He tried to hold her, but she kicked him in the shin. It seemed that everything he tried only served to aggravate her, so he withdrew to another room. She continued to yell and cry. He sobbed as he listened to her and felt so helpless. He wanted so much to comfort her but simply was at a loss on how to do so.

After about twenty minutes, she began to quiet down a little, though still whimpering softly. He came back to the room where she just stood looking at the wall. With tears still meandering down his cheeks, he softly whispered, "Betty Jo?" He waited for what her response might be. There was a brief pause, but then she turned to him and the lost gaze in her eyes showed some form of brightening recognition. She stepped toward William and burrowed her face into his chest as he wrapped his arms around her. She was silent and didn't move. William immediately began to weep silently as he held his beautiful wife in his arms. One of the hardest moments, but one of the most cherished. Though it didn't always happen, this time he was honored to have the opportunity to comfort this precious soul that he loved so dearly.

Chapter 21
Getting Close To Good-bye

Betty Jo's mental state hadn't changed much for a while, but physically, she was declining. Her gait was getting a little unsteady and she was having more difficulty swallowing. She ate like a bird and liked to walk around the house at night. William was exhausted and he didn't know how she did so much walking around the house at all hours without sleeping more than an hour or two here and there.

She was quite thin from not eating much and almost constantly walking. She had a couple of falls, but managed to only get some small bruises. One day while eating some chicken soup, her trouble with swallowing manifested itself. She coughed and sputtered a bit. It didn't seem that bad at the time, but a few hours later, she had a low-grade fever and actually chose to go to bed. She slept past her recent 1-2 hour stints. After about 5 hours of sleeping, William noticed some congestion in her breathing. He suspected she might have aspirated some of that soup into her lungs.

He could not get her to the doctor and didn't want to call the ambulance. He called her doctor who was also a friend, having known their family for many years. He told William he would come out after he was done with patients in the office. When he came out, he confirmed that she likely had aspiration pneumonia. He brought with him some antibiotic samples and left them with William along with a prescription. Betty Jo was hit and miss with taking oral medications, however, but William told the doctor he'd try all day as needed to make sure she got them down.

Betty Jo didn't wake up even during the exam. They opted to give her an intramuscular injection of Rocephin, an antibiotic to kick-start recovery. Even the shot didn't wake her up. William had this nagging thought in his spirit that this might be it, that she was not going to recover. He quickly dismissed it and thanked his friend for coming out. The doctor told him to call him if any other concerns arose or if Betty Jo was not cooperating consistently with taking the antibiotic and he would come back out.

Chapter 22
Showing Little Improvement

After the doctor's visit, Betty Jo slept a couple more hours before rustling and mumbling softly. William sat next to her and tried to converse with her, but she never woke up to full alertness. Not even alert enough to offer her water. He tried to elevate her a little higher by putting more pillows behind her, but then she would just turn over off the pillow. Her congestion was still present, but seemed like it might be a little bit better. William gave it another day, but it just didn't seem like she was continuing with any progress and he was only able to get occasional sips of water down her, but not her medication. He phoned the doctor who suggested she go to the hospital at this point or he'd be willing to come back out and give her another antibiotic injection.

William's soul was in anguish with the decisions he had to make. He still had that nagging thought too that this was Betty Jo's time to leave this current earth. He prayed and prayed for the wisdom to do what was right. He called his daughter Willa to let her know that her mom was not improving. He told her that he believed this might be her time. Willa had made arrangements to come home in a few days if her mom was not improving, but was able to bump those plans up.

William after much languishing knew Betty Jo was

suffering from this disease and if she recovered from this pneumonia, it would continue. He also knew that treating her aggressively in the hospital would not be something he thinks she would choose. He decided that he should give the second shot of antibiotic a chance. It could help her kick this pneumonia or maybe give him just a few more moments with his wife before he said good-bye. He called the doctor and he came out right away to give her another antibiotic injection and said he could come out daily if she is showing improvement.

Willa arrived home and he had her watch over her as he worked out in the barn. Willa wondered what he was doing as he would come back in the house briefly, then bring furniture out one by one, all at a meaningful pace. He brought a mattress out, some chairs, blankets, photos, space heaters and water pitcher. After a while, he came back in to check on her.

Betty Jo had briefly awoken, but not fully and seemed a little in distress when she rustled. He asked Willa if she was able to help him carry her to the barn if he lifted her upper body and she lifted her lower body? Willa, a little puzzled said she thought she could do that.

They carefully lifted her and took her out to the barn. William had cleaned and beautifully decorated one of the stalls. They gently laid her down on the mattress, which was on the ground, so the animals he brought into her could lay down next to her by the bed. He covered her up, then brought in one of his gentler cows and a sheep and tied them close to her bed. The farm had always been a comfort to her even as a child and he hoped that this would bring peace to her, either in her last moments on earth or in her recovery.

Willa hugged her dad, "what a tender gift you are giving her. You are amazing, Dad." William thanked Willa, "thank you, honey, I hope it is a gift that will help her."

Betty Jo woke up enough to notice she was not in her room anymore. She gazed around, then sighed and smiled. Then she nestled down into her pillows and closed her eyes. William rarely saw her smile since her Alzheimer's had moved into the more challenging stages. Just that brief smile triggered the waterworks and tears made their way from his eyes down his cheeks.

Their cow and sheep lay close to the bed with their heads resting on the bed. It was like they knew something was up. It was an hour later when Betty Jo woke up enough to interact. She was able to take a few sips of water and a few bites of ground-up meat, potatoes and gravy. William wasn't sure she fully recognized who he and Willa were, but it didn't seem to matter. She was calm, despite still having congestion in her breathing. It was helpful to have her sitting up, which they rarely had been able to do. Later William let the doctor know how she was doing and he came out again to give her an antibiotic injection.

It seemed odd, but for those few moments that she woke up in the barn, she seemed more at peace than she had been in a long, long time.

Chapter 23
The Last Embrace

The next day, following those few special moments of alertness in the barn, she began tossing and turning, her congestion worse and her facial expression distressed. She looked around the barn stall room like she was searching for something, then her eyes met William's. She cried out and William threw her arms around her quickly. She nestled her face into his chest and was quiet for what seemed like at least 15 minutes, then she slowly fell back into the bed and was unresponsive. Her breathing was still congested, but a little quieter. William knew this was the last embrace he would have with his wife until they were reunited in heaven.

The next couple of days, Betty Jo laid in her bed, sometimes very still, other times restless. William called in hospice to make sure she had what she needed to be comfortable. Over those two days, her breathing had changed and she did not wake up. It was time for her to go. For William, it was a bittersweet moment as he knew she would be off to a better place, but he would so miss her.

Her spirit given to her by the Almighty God would be free without the confines and limits of expression this earthly disease afflicted her with. He started thinking about her smile and laughter that would have an outlet again once in heaven. He smiled as he stared lovingly at her, but not without tears.

In an attempt to balance his anticipatory grief of not having her with him anymore, he imagined how happy she would be again once delivered safely to heaven. How wonderful that would be for her to be home with her Savior, Jesus. One cannot adequately describe what that must be like, but he pondered on the wonder of that impending experience for her.

He envisioned the giddy greetings that would probably take place as she was ushered into heaven. Her parents would be overjoyed to be with her again as well as her brother and sister. And his precious wife will be bubbling over with peace and ecstatic joy one can only endeavor to envision this side of heaven. She might miss her loved ones on earth, but she will have a heavenly perspective that gives her peace about that, a peace that we can't fully comprehend on earth. In other words though, William felt confident that she would be safe and happy.

His soul was aching though even though he knew their separation would only be temporary. Truly though, they will never be completely apart as their spirits were connected in love through their life together. Death cannot take that away as she lives on as her spirit vacates her current earthly body to move onto her new home. He knows he hasn't lost her as he knows where she will be. And she will be whole again and safe. He can focus on her joyful smiling face that she will have in heaven and not on the pain and difficulties she faced before her passing. A peace suddenly overwhelmed William as God's encouraging words flooded his spirit with a reassuring calm. It is like he buried his face into the word of God and he felt His reassuring embrace that it was going to be all right.

As he was contemplating all this in preparation, Betty Jo's respiration began to slow and be erratic with long periods of not breathing in between. William took her hand and laid his head next to it. He prayed quietly for her. He felt an ever so slight squeeze of his hand and as he looked up, she took her last breath. It was like he felt his wife leave her body and his presence, yet he also strangely felt that she was still with him. She would somehow always be part of him and be with him as their lives were entwined through the years together.

Willa tearfully said, "Good-bye Mom," and she and her dad hugged. They both knew she had successfully finished her pilgrimage through Alzheimer's to heaven and their new life chapter, as they wait to join her, had now begun.

Books by Tana Osborn

Until Heaven Then My Friend - Life's Journey For Your Beloved Dog

Turning Grief Into Sweet Memories

Passing - One Man's Pilgrimage Through Cancer To Heaven

Passing - One Woman's Pilgrimage Through Alzheimer's To Heaven

Passing – One Young Man's Pilgrimage Through Suicide To Heaven (Estimated availability December 2020)

Passing – A Woman's Pilgrimage Through Rebellion and Drug Overdose To Heaven (Estimated availability March 2021)

Finding Streams in the Wasteland - The Aftermath of Suicide and a Mother's Anguish (Estimated availability July 2021)

More books to come in the *Passing* series and related series.

Stay tuned @ www.tanaosborn.com/book-release-updates

Request for Review

☺

If you found this book to be helpful for you, I'd love to have you leave your thoughts on our review page. If you purchased this book on Amazon or other online retailer, you can go back to the book page and leave a review there. I would be so appreciative.

If you purchased the pdf copy from my website, please send your thoughts to me at lifesjourneytogether@gmail.com as I'd still love to know your thoughts. I can include your review on our detailed sales page for the book. You can be assured that I never use anyone's email on the book information or sales page nor share your email with anyone without permission.

Thank you so much for your purchase. I hope you did find encouragement in this novella about Betty Jo.

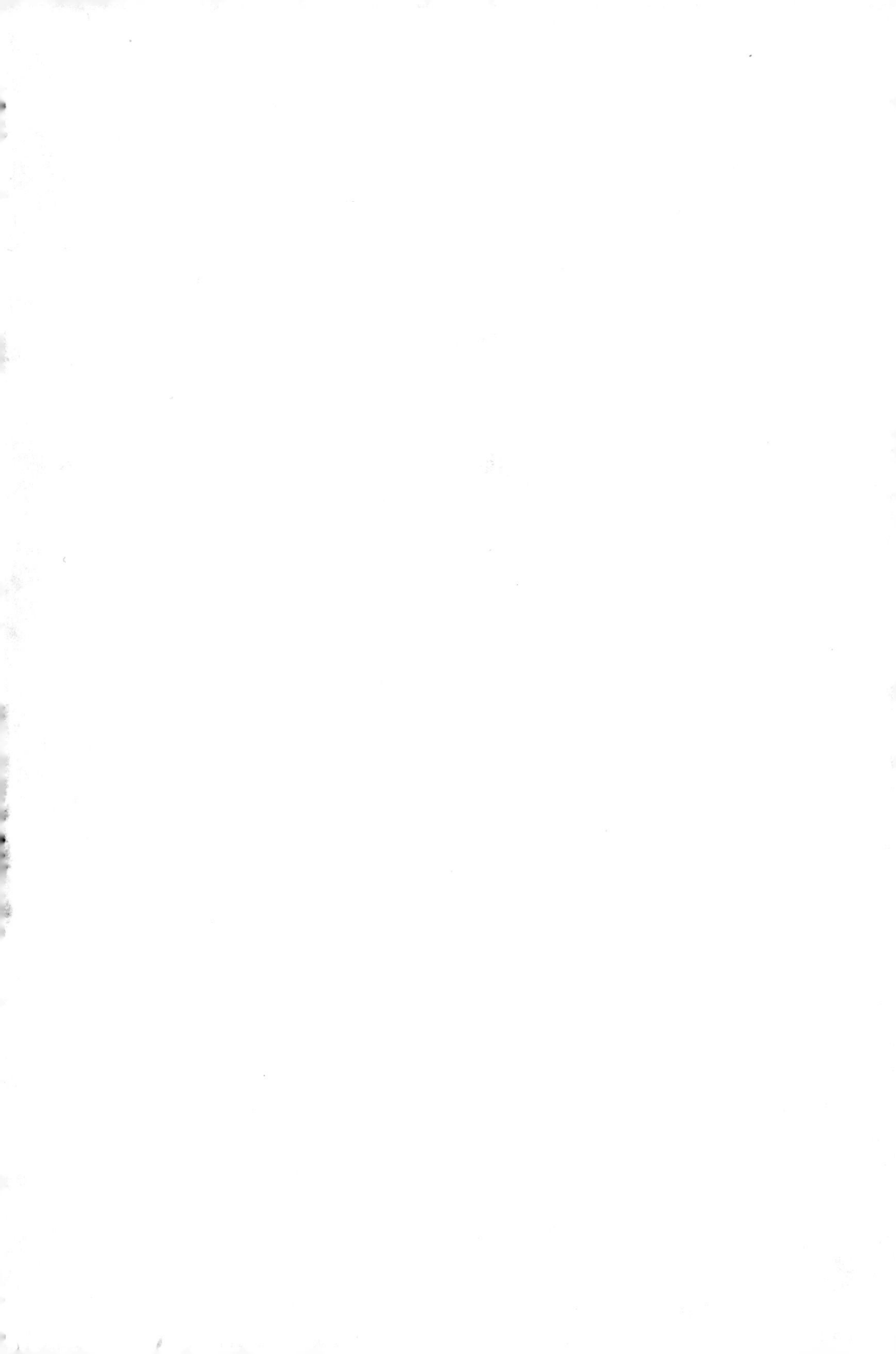